INTERMITTENT

FASTING

JOURNAL

This information is solely intended to provide assistance to you in your personal healthy eating efforts. The information is not intended as a substitute for consultation, evaluation or treatment by a medical professional and/or registered dietitian or nutritionist.

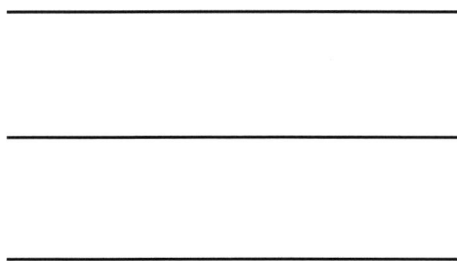

GOALS

Date					
	Goal	Day 1	Day 30	Day 60	Day 90 !
Weight					
Chest					
Waist					
Hips					
Thighs					
Arms					

Other Goals (energy level, cravings, digestion, skin ....)

_____

_____

_____

_____

_____

_____

_____

HUNGER LEVEL:
1 2 3 4 5 6 7 8 9 10

M T W T F S S

DATE: _____

WEIGHT: _____

DAY
1

Time	Food/Beverage	Calories

STARTED NEW FAST AT: _____ / NA   ENERGY LEVEL: 1 2 3 4 5 6 7 8 9 10

CHECK NUMBER OF 8 OZ
GLASSES OF WATER:

Time	Exercise	Amount

MOOD/CHALLENGES/NSV'S:

DAY 2

M T W T F S S

DATE: _____

WEIGHT: _____

HOURS FASTED BEFORE EATING: _____

HUNGER LEVEL:

1 2 3 4 5 6 7 8 9 10

Time	Food/Beverage	Calories

STARTED NEW FAST AT: _____ / NA   ENERGY LEVEL: 1 2 3 4 5 6 7 8 9 10

CHECK NUMBER OF 8 OZ
GLASSES OF WATER:

Time	Exercise	Amount

MOOD/CHALLENGES/NSV'S:

_____

_____

_____

HOURS FASTED BEFORE EATING: _____

HUNGER LEVEL:
1 2 3 4 5 6 7 8 9 10

M T W T F S S

DATE: _____

WEIGHT: _____

DAY
3

Time	Food/Beverage	Calories

STARTED NEW FAST AT: _____/ NA   ENERGY LEVEL: 1 2 3 4 5 6 7 8 9 10

CHECK NUMBER OF 8 OZ
GLASSES OF WATER:

Time	Exercise	Amount

MOOD/CHALLENGES/NSV'S: _____
_____
_____
_____

<table>
<tr><td>**DAY**
4</td><td>M T W T F S S

DATE: _____

WEIGHT: _____</td><td>HOURS FASTED BEFORE EATING: _____

HUNGER LEVEL:
1 2 3 4 5 6 7 8 9 10</td></tr>
</table>

Time	Food/Beverage	Calories

STARTED NEW FAST AT: _____ / NA   ENERGY LEVEL: 1 2 3 4 5 6 7 8 9 10

CHECK NUMBER OF 8 OZ GLASSES OF WATER:

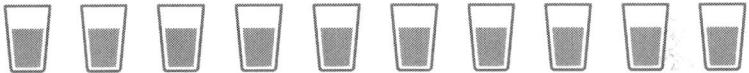

Time	Exercise	Amount

MOOD/CHALLENGES/NSV'S:

_____

_____

_____

_____

HOURS FASTED BEFORE EATING: _____

HUNGER LEVEL:
1 2 3 4 5 6 7 8 9 10

M T W T F S S

DATE: _____

WEIGHT: _____

DAY
5

Time	Food/Beverage	Calories

STARTED NEW FAST AT: _____ / NA   ENERGY LEVEL: 1 2 3 4 5 6 7 8 9 10

CHECK NUMBER OF 8 OZ
GLASSES OF WATER:

Time	Exercise	Amount

MOOD/CHALLENGES/NSV'S: _____

_____

_____

DAY 6	M T W T F S S DATE: _____ WEIGHT: _____	HOURS FASTED BEFORE EATING: _____ HUNGER LEVEL: 1 2 3 4 5 6 7 8 9 10

Time	Food/Beverage	Calories

STARTED NEW FAST AT: _____/ NA   ENERGY LEVEL: 1 2 3 4 5 6 7 8 9 10

CHECK NUMBER OF 8 OZ GLASSES OF WATER:

Time	Exercise	Amount

MOOD/CHALLENGES/NSV'S:

_____

_____

_____

_____

HOURS FASTED BEFORE EATING: _____

HUNGER LEVEL:

1 2 3 4 5 6 7 8 9 10

M T W T F S S

DATE: _____

WEIGHT: _____

DAY
7

Time	Food/Beverage	Calories

STARTED NEW FAST AT: _____ / NA   ENERGY LEVEL: 1 2 3 4 5 6 7 8 9 10

CHECK NUMBER OF 8 OZ
GLASSES OF WATER:

Time	Exercise	Amount

MOOD/CHALLENGES/NSV'S: _____

DAY 8

M T W T F S S

DATE: _____

WEIGHT: _____

Time	Food/Beverage	Calories

STARTED NEW FAST AT: _____/ NA   ENERGY LEVEL: 1 2 3 4 5 6 7 8 9 10

CHECK NUMBER OF 8 OZ
GLASSES OF WATER:

Time	Exercise	Amount

MOOD/CHALLENGES/NSV'S:

HOURS FASTED BEFORE EATING: _____

HUNGER LEVEL:

1 2 3 4 5 6 7 8 9 10

M T W T F S S

DATE: _____

WEIGHT: _____

Time	Food/Beverage	Calories

STARTED NEW FAST AT: _____/ NA   ENERGY LEVEL: 1 2 3 4 5 6 7 8 9 10

CHECK NUMBER OF 8 OZ
GLASSES OF WATER:

Time	Exercise	Amount

MOOD/CHALLENGES/NSV'S:

_____

_____

_____

_____

| DAY 10 | M T W T F S S Date: _____ weight: _____ | Hours fasted before eating: _____ Hunger level: 1 2 3 4 5 6 7 8 9 10 |

Time	Food/Beverage	Calories

STARTED NEW FAST AT: _____ / NA   ENERGY LEVEL: 1 2 3 4 5 6 7 8 9 10

CHECK NUMBER OF 8 OZ GLASSES OF WATER:

Time	Exercise	Amount

MOOD/CHALLENGES/NSV'S:
_____
_____
_____
_____

HOURS FASTED BEFORE EATING: _____	M T W T F S S	DAY
HUNGER LEVEL:	DATE: _____	11
1 2 3 4 5 6 7 8 9 10	WEIGHT: _____	

Time	Food/Beverage	Calories

STARTED NEW FAST AT: _____ / NA   ENERGY LEVEL: 1 2 3 4 5 6 7 8 9 10

CHECK NUMBER OF 8 OZ GLASSES OF WATER:

Time	Exercise	Amount

MOOD/CHALLENGES/NSV'S: _____
_____
_____
_____

DAY 12

M T W T F S S

Date: _____

Weight: _____

Time	Food/Beverage	Calories

STARTED NEW FAST AT: _____ / NA   ENERGY LEVEL: 1 2 3 4 5 6 7 8 9 10

CHECK NUMBER OF 8 OZ GLASSES OF WATER:

Time	Exercise	Amount

MOOD/CHALLENGES/NSV'S:

_____

_____

_____

_____

HOURS FASTED BEFORE EATING: _____

HUNGER LEVEL:

1 2 3 4 5 6 7 8 9 10

M T W T F S S

DATE: _____

WEIGHT: _____

DAY 13

Time	Food/Beverage	Calories

STARTED NEW FAST AT: _____/ NA   ENERGY LEVEL: 1 2 3 4 5 6 7 8 9 10

CHECK NUMBER OF 8 OZ GLASSES OF WATER:

Time	Exercise	Amount

MOOD/CHALLENGES/NSV'S: _____

_____

_____

_____

<table>
<tr><td rowspan="3">DAY
14</td><td>M T W T F S S</td><td>HOURS FASTED BEFORE EATING: _____</td></tr>
<tr><td>DATE: _____</td><td rowspan="2">HUNGER LEVEL:
1 2 3 4 5 6 7 8 9 10</td></tr>
<tr><td>WEIGHT: _____</td></tr>
</table>

Time	Food/Beverage	Calories

STARTED NEW FAST AT: _____ / NA   ENERGY LEVEL: 1 2 3 4 5 6 7 8 9 10

CHECK NUMBER OF 8 OZ GLASSES OF WATER:

Time	Exercise	Amount

MOOD/CHALLENGES/NSV'S:
_____
_____
_____
_____

HOURS FASTED BEFORE EATING: _____

HUNGER LEVEL:

1 2 3 4 5 6 7 8 9 10

M T W T F S S

DATE: _____

WEIGHT: _____

Time	Food/Beverage	Calories

STARTED NEW FAST AT: _____ / NA   ENERGY LEVEL: 1 2 3 4 5 6 7 8 9 10

CHECK NUMBER OF 8 OZ
GLASSES OF WATER:

Time	Exercise	Amount

MOOD/CHALLENGES/NSV'S: _____

_____

_____

_____

DAY 16

M T W T F S S

Date: _____

Weight: _____

HOURS FASTED BEFORE EATING: _____

HUNGER LEVEL:
1 2 3 4 5 6 7 8 9 10

Time	Food/Beverage	Calories

STARTED NEW FAST AT: _____ / NA   ENERGY LEVEL: 1 2 3 4 5 6 7 8 9 10

CHECK NUMBER OF 8 OZ GLASSES OF WATER:

Time	Exercise	Amount

MOOD/CHALLENGES/NSV'S:

_____
_____
_____
_____

HOURS FASTED BEFORE EATING: _____

HUNGER LEVEL:
1 2 3 4 5 6 7 8 9 10

M T W T F S S

DATE: _____

WEIGHT: _____

DAY 17

Time	Food/Beverage	Calories

STARTED NEW FAST AT: _____ / NA   ENERGY LEVEL: 1 2 3 4 5 6 7 8 9 10

CHECK NUMBER OF 8 OZ GLASSES OF WATER:

Time	Exercise	Amount

MOOD/CHALLENGES/NSV'S: _____

_____

_____

_____

<table>
<tr><td rowspan="3">DAY
18</td><td>M T W T F S S</td><td>HOURS FASTED BEFORE EATING: _____</td></tr>
<tr><td>DATE: _____</td><td rowspan="2">HUNGER LEVEL:
1 2 3 4 5 6 7 8 9 10</td></tr>
<tr><td>WEIGHT: _____</td></tr>
</table>

Time	Food/Beverage	Calories

STARTED NEW FAST AT: _____ / NA   ENERGY LEVEL: 1 2 3 4 5 6 7 8 9 10

CHECK NUMBER OF 8 OZ GLASSES OF WATER:

Time	Exercise	Amount

MOOD/CHALLENGES/NSV'S:

_____
_____
_____
_____

HOURS FASTED BEFORE EATING: _____

HUNGER LEVEL:
1 2 3 4 5 6 7 8 9 10

M T W T F S S

DATE: _____

WEIGHT: _____

Time	Food/Beverage	Calories

STARTED NEW FAST AT: _____/ NA   ENERGY LEVEL: 1 2 3 4 5 6 7 8 9 10

CHECK NUMBER OF 8 OZ
GLASSES OF WATER:

Time	Exercise	Amount

MOOD/CHALLENGES/NSV'S: _____
_____
_____
_____

DAY 20	M T W T F S S DATE: _____ WEIGHT: _____	HOURS FASTED BEFORE EATING: _____ HUNGER LEVEL: 1 2 3 4 5 6 7 8 9 10

Time	Food/Beverage	Calories

STARTED NEW FAST AT: _____ / NA   ENERGY LEVEL: 1 2 3 4 5 6 7 8 9 10

CHECK NUMBER OF 8 OZ
GLASSES OF WATER:

Time	Exercise	Amount

MOOD/CHALLENGES/NSV'S:

HOURS FASTED BEFORE EATING: _____

HUNGER LEVEL:
1 2 3 4 5 6 7 8 9 10

M T W T F S S

DATE: _____

WEIGHT: _____

DAY
21

Time	Food/Beverage	Calories

STARTED NEW FAST AT: _____/ NA   ENERGY LEVEL: 1 2 3 4 5 6 7 8 9 10

CHECK NUMBER OF 8 OZ
GLASSES OF WATER:

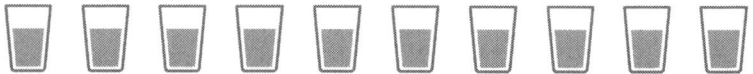

Time	Exercise	Amount

MOOD/CHALLENGES/NSV'S: _____

_____

_____

_____

<table>
<tr><td rowspan="3">**DAY**
22</td><td>M T W T F S S</td><td>HOURS FASTED BEFORE EATING: _____</td></tr>
<tr><td>DATE: _____</td><td>HUNGER LEVEL:</td></tr>
<tr><td>WEIGHT: _____</td><td>1 2 3 4 5 6 7 8 9 10</td></tr>
</table>

Time	Food/Beverage	Calories

STARTED NEW FAST AT: _____ / NA   ENERGY LEVEL: 1 2 3 4 5 6 7 8 9 10

CHECK NUMBER OF 8 OZ
GLASSES OF WATER:

Time	Exercise	Amount

MOOD/CHALLENGES/NSV'S:

_____
_____
_____
_____

HOURS FASTED BEFORE EATING: _____

HUNGER LEVEL:
1 2 3 4 5 6 7 8 9 10

M T W T F S S

DATE: _____

WEIGHT: _____

DAY
23

Time	Food/Beverage	Calories

STARTED NEW FAST AT: _____ / NA   ENERGY LEVEL: 1 2 3 4 5 6 7 8 9 10

CHECK NUMBER OF 8 OZ
GLASSES OF WATER:

Time	Exercise	Amount

MOOD/CHALLENGES/NSV'S: _____
_____
_____
_____

DAY 24

M T W T F S S

DATE: _____

WEIGHT: _____

HOURS FASTED BEFORE EATING: _____

HUNGER LEVEL:
1 2 3 4 5 6 7 8 9 10

Time	Food/Beverage	Calories

STARTED NEW FAST AT: _____ / NA   ENERGY LEVEL: 1 2 3 4 5 6 7 8 9 10

CHECK NUMBER OF 8 OZ GLASSES OF WATER:

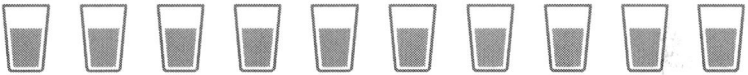

Time	Exercise	Amount

MOOD/CHALLENGES/NSV'S:

HOURS FASTED BEFORE EATING: _____

HUNGER LEVEL:
1 2 3 4 5 6 7 8 9 10

M T W T F S S

DATE: _____

WEIGHT: _____

DAY 25

Time	Food/Beverage	Calories

STARTED NEW FAST AT: _____ / NA   ENERGY LEVEL: 1 2 3 4 5 6 7 8 9 10

CHECK NUMBER OF 8 OZ GLASSES OF WATER:

Time	Exercise	Amount

MOOD/CHALLENGES/NSV'S:
_____
_____
_____
_____

<table>
<tr><td colspan="2">

DAY
26

</td><td>

M T W T F S S

DATE: _____

WEIGHT: _____

</td><td>

</td></tr>
</table>

Time	Food/Beverage	Calories

STARTED NEW FAST AT: _____ / NA   ENERGY LEVEL: 1 2 3 4 5 6 7 8 9 10

CHECK NUMBER OF 8 OZ
GLASSES OF WATER:

Time	Exercise	Amount

MOOD/CHALLENGES/NSV'S:

_____

_____

_____

_____

HOURS FASTED BEFORE EATING: _____

HUNGER LEVEL:
1 2 3 4 5 6 7 8 9 10

M T W T F S S

DATE: _____

WEIGHT: _____

DAY
27

Time	Food/Beverage	Calories

STARTED NEW FAST AT: _____ / NA   ENERGY LEVEL: 1 2 3 4 5 6 7 8 9 10

CHECK NUMBER OF 8 OZ
GLASSES OF WATER:

Time	Exercise	Amount

MOOD/CHALLENGES/NSV'S:

_____

_____

_____

| DAY 28 | M T W T F S S Date: _____ Weight: _____ | Hours Fasted Before Eating: _____ Hunger Level: 1 2 3 4 5 6 7 8 9 10 |

Time	Food/Beverage	Calories

Started New Fast At: _____ / NA   Energy Level: 1 2 3 4 5 6 7 8 9 10

Check Number of 8 oz Glasses of Water:

Time	Exercise	Amount

Mood/Challenges/NSV's: _____
_____
_____
_____

HOURS FASTED BEFORE EATING: _____

HUNGER LEVEL:

1 2 3 4 5 6 7 8 9 10

M T W T F S S

DATE: _____

WEIGHT: _____

DAY
29

Time	Food/Beverage	Calories

STARTED NEW FAST AT: _____ / NA   ENERGY LEVEL: 1 2 3 4 5 6 7 8 9 10

CHECK NUMBER OF 8 OZ
GLASSES OF WATER:

Time	Exercise	Amount

MOOD/CHALLENGES/NSV'S:

DAY 30

M T W T F S S

DATE: _____

WEIGHT: _____

HOURS FASTED BEFORE EATING: _____

HUNGER LEVEL:
1 2 3 4 5 6 7 8 9 10

Time	Food/Beverage	Calories

STARTED NEW FAST AT: _____ / NA   ENERGY LEVEL: 1 2 3 4 5 6 7 8 9 10

CHECK NUMBER OF 8 OZ GLASSES OF WATER:

Time	Exercise	Amount

MOOD/CHALLENGES/NSV'S: _____

HOURS FASTED BEFORE EATING: _____

HUNGER LEVEL:

1 2 3 4 5 6 7 8 9 10

M T W T F S S

DATE: _____

WEIGHT: _____

DAY
31

Time	Food/Beverage	Calories

STARTED NEW FAST AT: _____/ NA   ENERGY LEVEL: 1 2 3 4 5 6 7 8 9 10

CHECK NUMBER OF 8 OZ
GLASSES OF WATER:

Time	Exercise	Amount

MOOD/CHALLENGES/NSV'S: _____

_____

_____

_____

DAY	M T W T F S S	HOURS FASTED BEFORE EATING: _____
32	DATE: _____	HUNGER LEVEL:
	WEIGHT: _____	1 2 3 4 5 6 7 8 9 10

Time	Food/Beverage	Calories

STARTED NEW FAST AT: _____ / NA   ENERGY LEVEL: 1 2 3 4 5 6 7 8 9 10

CHECK NUMBER OF 8 OZ GLASSES OF WATER:

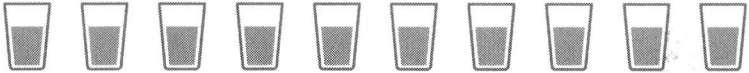

Time	Exercise	Amount

MOOD/CHALLENGES/NSV'S:

_____

_____

_____

_____

HOURS FASTED BEFORE EATING: _____

HUNGER LEVEL:

1 2 3 4 5 6 7 8 9 10

M T W T F S S

DATE: _____

WEIGHT: _____

Time	Food/Beverage	Calories

STARTED NEW FAST AT: _____ / NA   ENERGY LEVEL: 1 2 3 4 5 6 7 8 9 10

CHECK NUMBER OF 8 OZ
GLASSES OF WATER:

Time	Exercise	Amount

MOOD/CHALLENGES/NSV'S:

_____

_____

_____

DAY 34	M T W T F S S DATE: _____ WEIGHT: _____	HOURS FASTED BEFORE EATING: _____ HUNGER LEVEL: 1 2 3 4 5 6 7 8 9 10

Time	Food/Beverage	Calories

STARTED NEW FAST AT: _____ / NA   ENERGY LEVEL: 1 2 3 4 5 6 7 8 9 10

CHECK NUMBER OF 8 OZ GLASSES OF WATER:

Time	Exercise	Amount

MOOD/CHALLENGES/NSV'S:
_____
_____
_____
_____

HOURS FASTED BEFORE EATING: _____

HUNGER LEVEL:
1 2 3 4 5 6 7 8 9 10

M T W T F S S

DATE: _____

WEIGHT: _____

DAY
35

Time	Food/Beverage	Calories

STARTED NEW FAST AT: _____ / NA   ENERGY LEVEL: 1 2 3 4 5 6 7 8 9 10

CHECK NUMBER OF 8 OZ
GLASSES OF WATER:

Time	Exercise	Amount

MOOD/CHALLENGES/NSV'S: _____

_____

_____

_____

DAY 36	M T W T F S S	HOURS FASTED BEFORE EATING: _____
	DATE: _____	HUNGER LEVEL:
	WEIGHT: _____	1 2 3 4 5 6 7 8 9 10

Time	Food/Beverage	Calories

STARTED NEW FAST AT: _____ / NA   ENERGY LEVEL: 1 2 3 4 5 6 7 8 9 10

CHECK NUMBER OF 8 OZ GLASSES OF WATER:

Time	Exercise	Amount

MOOD/CHALLENGES/NSV'S:
_____
_____
_____
_____

HOURS FASTED BEFORE EATING: _____

HUNGER LEVEL:
1 2 3 4 5 6 7 8 9 10

M T W T F S S

DATE: _____

WEIGHT: _____

DAY
37

Time	Food/Beverage	Calories

STARTED NEW FAST AT: _____/ NA   ENERGY LEVEL: 1 2 3 4 5 6 7 8 9 10

CHECK NUMBER OF 8 OZ
GLASSES OF WATER:

Time	Exercise	Amount

MOOD/CHALLENGES/NSV'S: _____

_____

_____

_____

DAY 38	M T W T F S S DATE: _____ WEIGHT: _____	HOURS FASTED BEFORE EATING: _____ HUNGER LEVEL: 1 2 3 4 5 6 7 8 9 10

Time	Food/Beverage	Calories

STARTED NEW FAST AT: _____ / NA   ENERGY LEVEL: 1 2 3 4 5 6 7 8 9 10

CHECK NUMBER OF 8 OZ GLASSES OF WATER:

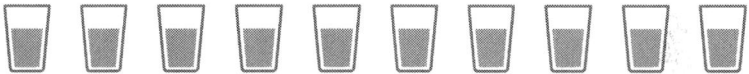

Time	Exercise	Amount

MOOD/CHALLENGES/NSV'S:

_____

_____

_____

_____

HOURS FASTED BEFORE EATING: _____

HUNGER LEVEL:
1 2 3 4 5 6 7 8 9 10

M T W T F S S

DATE: _____

WEIGHT: _____

DAY 39

Time	Food/Beverage	Calories

STARTED NEW FAST AT: _____/ NA   ENERGY LEVEL: 1 2 3 4 5 6 7 8 9 10

CHECK NUMBER OF 8 OZ GLASSES OF WATER:

Time	Exercise	Amount

MOOD/CHALLENGES/NSV'S: _____

_____

_____

_____

DAY 40

M T W T F S S

DATE: _____

WEIGHT: _____

HOURS FASTED BEFORE EATING: _____

HUNGER LEVEL:

1 2 3 4 5 6 7 8 9 10

Time	Food/Beverage	Calories

STARTED NEW FAST AT: _____ / NA   ENERGY LEVEL: 1 2 3 4 5 6 7 8 9 10

CHECK NUMBER OF 8 OZ GLASSES OF WATER:

Time	Exercise	Amount

MOOD/CHALLENGES/NSV'S:

_____

_____

_____

HOURS FASTED BEFORE EATING: _____

HUNGER LEVEL:
1 2 3 4 5 6 7 8 9 10

M T W T F S S

DATE: _____

WEIGHT: _____

Time	Food/Beverage	Calories

STARTED NEW FAST AT: _____/ NA   ENERGY LEVEL: 1 2 3 4 5 6 7 8 9 10

CHECK NUMBER OF 8 OZ
GLASSES OF WATER:

Time	Exercise	Amount

MOOD/CHALLENGES/NSV'S:

_____

_____

_____

_____

DAY	M T W T F S S	HOURS FASTED BEFORE EATING: _____
42	DATE: _____	HUNGER LEVEL:
	WEIGHT: _____	1 2 3 4 5 6 7 8 9 10

Time	Food/Beverage	Calories

STARTED NEW FAST AT: _____ / NA   ENERGY LEVEL: 1 2 3 4 5 6 7 8 9 10

CHECK NUMBER OF 8 OZ GLASSES OF WATER:

Time	Exercise	Amount

MOOD/CHALLENGES/NSV'S:

_____

_____

_____

HOURS FASTED BEFORE EATING: _____

HUNGER LEVEL:

1 2 3 4 5 6 7 8 9 10

M T W T F S S

DATE: _____

WEIGHT: _____

DAY
43

Time	Food/Beverage	Calories

STARTED NEW FAST AT: _____/ NA   ENERGY LEVEL: 1 2 3 4 5 6 7 8 9 10

CHECK NUMBER OF 8 OZ
GLASSES OF WATER:

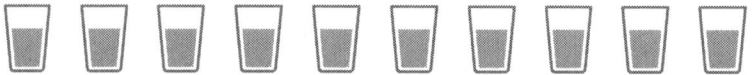

Time	Exercise	Amount

MOOD/CHALLENGES/NSV'S:

_____

_____

_____

DAY 44

M T W T F S S

DATE: _____

WEIGHT: _____

HOURS FASTED BEFORE EATING: _____

HUNGER LEVEL:

1 2 3 4 5 6 7 8 9 10

Time	Food/Beverage	Calories

STARTED NEW FAST AT: _____ / NA   ENERGY LEVEL: 1 2 3 4 5 6 7 8 9 10

CHECK NUMBER OF 8 OZ GLASSES OF WATER:

Time	Exercise	Amount

MOOD/CHALLENGES/NSV'S:

HOURS FASTED BEFORE EATING: _____

M T W T F S S

DATE: _____

WEIGHT: _____

DAY 45

HUNGER LEVEL:

1 2 3 4 5 6 7 8 9 10

Time	Food/Beverage	Calories

STARTED NEW FAST AT: _____/ NA   ENERGY LEVEL: 1 2 3 4 5 6 7 8 9 10

CHECK NUMBER OF 8 OZ
GLASSES OF WATER:

Time	Exercise	Amount

MOOD/CHALLENGES/NSV'S: _____

_____

_____

_____

DAY 46	M T W T F S S DATE: _____ WEIGHT: _____	HOURS FASTED BEFORE EATING: _____ HUNGER LEVEL: 1 2 3 4 5 6 7 8 9 10

Time	Food/Beverage	Calories

STARTED NEW FAST AT: _____ / NA   ENERGY LEVEL: 1 2 3 4 5 6 7 8 9 10

CHECK NUMBER OF 8 OZ GLASSES OF WATER:

Time	Exercise	Amount

MOOD/CHALLENGES/NSV'S:
_____
_____
_____
_____

HOURS FASTED BEFORE EATING: _____

HUNGER LEVEL:

1 2 3 4 5 6 7 8 9 10

M T W T F S S

DATE: _____

WEIGHT: _____

Time	Food/Beverage	Calories

STARTED NEW FAST AT: _____/ NA   ENERGY LEVEL: 1 2 3 4 5 6 7 8 9 10

CHECK NUMBER OF 8 OZ
GLASSES OF WATER:

Time	Exercise	Amount

MOOD/CHALLENGES/NSV'S:

_____

_____

_____

DAY 48

M T W T F S S

DATE: _____

WEIGHT: _____

HOURS FASTED BEFORE EATING: _____

HUNGER LEVEL:

1 2 3 4 5 6 7 8 9 10

Time	Food/Beverage	Calories

STARTED NEW FAST AT: _____ / NA   ENERGY LEVEL: 1 2 3 4 5 6 7 8 9 10

CHECK NUMBER OF 8 OZ GLASSES OF WATER:

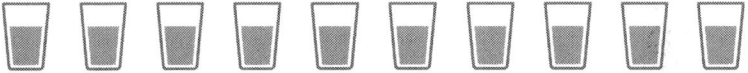

Time	Exercise	Amount

MOOD/CHALLENGES/NSV'S:

_____

_____

_____

HOURS FASTED BEFORE EATING: _____

HUNGER LEVEL:
1 2 3 4 5 6 7 8 9 10

M T W T F S S

DATE: _____

WEIGHT: _____

Time	Food/Beverage	Calories

STARTED NEW FAST AT: _____/ NA   ENERGY LEVEL: 1 2 3 4 5 6 7 8 9 10

CHECK NUMBER OF 8 OZ
GLASSES OF WATER:

Time	Exercise	Amount

MOOD/CHALLENGES/NSV'S:

_____

_____

_____

DAY 50

M T W T F S S

DATE: _____

WEIGHT: _____

HOURS FASTED BEFORE EATING: _____

HUNGER LEVEL:
1 2 3 4 5 6 7 8 9 10

Time	Food/Beverage	Calories

STARTED NEW FAST AT: _____ / NA   ENERGY LEVEL: 1 2 3 4 5 6 7 8 9 10

CHECK NUMBER OF 8 OZ GLASSES OF WATER:

Time	Exercise	Amount

MOOD/CHALLENGES/NSV'S:
_____
_____
_____
_____

HOURS FASTED BEFORE EATING: _____

HUNGER LEVEL:
1 2 3 4 5 6 7 8 9 10

M T W T F S S

DATE: _____

WEIGHT: _____

DAY
51

Time	Food/Beverage	Calories

STARTED NEW FAST AT: _____ / NA   ENERGY LEVEL: 1 2 3 4 5 6 7 8 9 10

CHECK NUMBER OF 8 OZ
GLASSES OF WATER:

Time	Exercise	Amount

MOOD/CHALLENGES/NSV'S: _____

_____

_____

_____

DAY
52

M T W T F S S

Date: _____

Weight: _____

HOURS FASTED BEFORE EATING: _____

HUNGER LEVEL:

1 2 3 4 5 6 7 8 9 10

Time	Food/Beverage	Calories

STARTED NEW FAST AT: _____ / NA   ENERGY LEVEL: 1 2 3 4 5 6 7 8 9 10

CHECK NUMBER OF 8 OZ
GLASSES OF WATER:

Time	Exercise	Amount

MOOD/CHALLENGES/NSV'S:

_____
_____
_____
_____

HOURS FASTED BEFORE EATING: _____

HUNGER LEVEL:
1 2 3 4 5 6 7 8 9 10

M T W T F S S

DATE: _____

WEIGHT: _____

DAY
53

Time	Food/Beverage	Calories

STARTED NEW FAST AT: _____ / NA   ENERGY LEVEL: 1 2 3 4 5 6 7 8 9 10

CHECK NUMBER OF 8 OZ
GLASSES OF WATER:

Time	Exercise	Amount

MOOD/CHALLENGES/NSV'S: _____

_____

_____

_____

DAY 54

M T W T F S S

DATE: _____

WEIGHT: _____

HOURS FASTED BEFORE EATING: _____

HUNGER LEVEL:
1 2 3 4 5 6 7 8 9 10

Time	Food/Beverage	Calories

STARTED NEW FAST AT: _____ / NA   ENERGY LEVEL: 1 2 3 4 5 6 7 8 9 10

CHECK NUMBER OF 8 OZ GLASSES OF WATER:

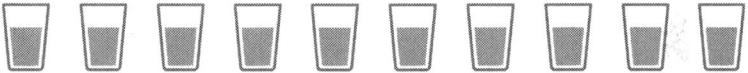

Time	Exercise	Amount

MOOD/CHALLENGES/NSV'S: _____
_____
_____
_____

HOURS FASTED BEFORE EATING: _____

HUNGER LEVEL:
1 2 3 4 5 6 7 8 9 10

M T W T F S S

DATE: _____

WEIGHT: _____

DAY 55

Time	Food/Beverage	Calories

STARTED NEW FAST AT: _____/ NA   ENERGY LEVEL: 1 2 3 4 5 6 7 8 9 10

CHECK NUMBER OF 8 OZ GLASSES OF WATER:

Time	Exercise	Amount

MOOD/CHALLENGES/NSV'S: _____
_____
_____
_____

DAY 56	M T W T F S S DATE: _____ WEIGHT: _____	HOURS FASTED BEFORE EATING: _____ HUNGER LEVEL: 1 2 3 4 5 6 7 8 9 10

Time	Food/Beverage	Calories

STARTED NEW FAST AT: _____ / NA   ENERGY LEVEL: 1 2 3 4 5 6 7 8 9 10

CHECK NUMBER OF 8 OZ
GLASSES OF WATER:

Time	Exercise	Amount

MOOD/CHALLENGES/NSV'S:

HOURS FASTED BEFORE EATING: _____	M T W T F S S	DAY
HUNGER LEVEL:	DATE: _____	57
1 2 3 4 5 6 7 8 9 10	WEIGHT: _____	

Time	Food/Beverage	Calories

STARTED NEW FAST AT: _____ / NA   ENERGY LEVEL: 1 2 3 4 5 6 7 8 9 10

CHECK NUMBER OF 8 OZ
GLASSES OF WATER:

Time	Exercise	Amount

MOOD/CHALLENGES/NSV'S: _____

_____

_____

_____

DAY 58	M T W T F S S DATE: _____ WEIGHT: _____	HOURS FASTED BEFORE EATING: _____ HUNGER LEVEL: 1 2 3 4 5 6 7 8 9 10

Time	Food/Beverage	Calories

STARTED NEW FAST AT: _____ / NA   ENERGY LEVEL: 1 2 3 4 5 6 7 8 9 10

CHECK NUMBER OF 8 OZ GLASSES OF WATER:

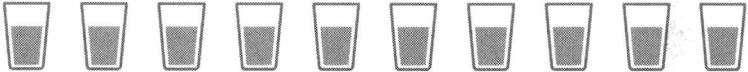

Time	Exercise	Amount

MOOD/CHALLENGES/NSV'S:

_____
_____
_____
_____

HOURS FASTED BEFORE EATING: _____

HUNGER LEVEL:

1 2 3 4 5 6 7 8 9 10

M T W T F S S

DATE: _____

WEIGHT: _____

DAY 59

Time	Food/Beverage	Calories

STARTED NEW FAST AT: _____ / NA   ENERGY LEVEL: 1 2 3 4 5 6 7 8 9 10

CHECK NUMBER OF 8 OZ GLASSES OF WATER:

Time	Exercise	Amount

MOOD/CHALLENGES/NSV'S: _____

_____

_____

_____

DAY 60

M T W T F S S

DATE: _____

WEIGHT: _____

HOURS FASTED BEFORE EATING: _____

HUNGER LEVEL:
1 2 3 4 5 6 7 8 9 10

Time	Food/Beverage	Calories

STARTED NEW FAST AT: _____/ NA   ENERGY LEVEL: 1 2 3 4 5 6 7 8 9 10

CHECK NUMBER OF 8 OZ
GLASSES OF WATER:

Time	Exercise	Amount

MOOD/CHALLENGES/NSV'S:

HOURS FASTED BEFORE EATING: _____		M T W T F S S		DAY
HUNGER LEVEL:		DATE: _____		61
1 2 3 4 5 6 7 8 9 10		WEIGHT: _____		

Time	Food/Beverage	Calories

STARTED NEW FAST AT: _____ / NA   ENERGY LEVEL: 1 2 3 4 5 6 7 8 9 10

CHECK NUMBER OF 8 OZ
GLASSES OF WATER:

Time	Exercise	Amount

MOOD/CHALLENGES/NSV'S: _____

_____

_____

_____

DAY 62

M T W T F S S

Date: _____

Weight: _____

Hours fasted before eating: _____

Hunger level:

1 2 3 4 5 6 7 8 9 10

Time	Food/Beverage	Calories

Started new fast at: _____/ NA   Energy level: 1 2 3 4 5 6 7 8 9 10

Check number of 8 oz glasses of water:

Time	Exercise	Amount

Mood/Challenges/NSV's:

_____

_____

_____

HOURS FASTED BEFORE EATING: _____

HUNGER LEVEL:
1 2 3 4 5 6 7 8 9 10

M T W T F S S

DATE: _____

WEIGHT: _____

DAY
63

Time	Food/Beverage	Calories

STARTED NEW FAST AT: _____ / NA   ENERGY LEVEL: 1 2 3 4 5 6 7 8 9 10

CHECK NUMBER OF 8 OZ
GLASSES OF WATER:

Time	Exercise	Amount

MOOD/CHALLENGES/NSV'S: _____

_____

_____

_____

DAY	M T W T F S S	HOURS FASTED BEFORE EATING: _____
64	DATE: _____	HUNGER LEVEL:
	WEIGHT: _____	1 2 3 4 5 6 7 8 9 10

Time	Food/Beverage	Calories

STARTED NEW FAST AT: _____ / NA   ENERGY LEVEL: 1 2 3 4 5 6 7 8 9 10

CHECK NUMBER OF 8 OZ GLASSES OF WATER:

Time	Exercise	Amount

MOOD/CHALLENGES/NSV'S:

_____

_____

_____

HOURS FASTED BEFORE EATING: _____

HUNGER LEVEL:

1 2 3 4 5 6 7 8 9 10

M T W T F S S

DATE: _____

WEIGHT: _____

DAY
65

Time	Food/Beverage	Calories

STARTED NEW FAST AT: _____/ NA   ENERGY LEVEL: 1 2 3 4 5 6 7 8 9 10

CHECK NUMBER OF 8 OZ
GLASSES OF WATER:

Time	Exercise	Amount

MOOD/CHALLENGES/NSV'S: _____

_____

_____

_____

DAY	M T W T F S S	HOURS FASTED BEFORE EATING: _____
66	DATE: _____	HUNGER LEVEL:
	WEIGHT: _____	1 2 3 4 5 6 7 8 9 10

Time	Food/Beverage	Calories

STARTED NEW FAST AT: _____ / NA   ENERGY LEVEL: 1 2 3 4 5 6 7 8 9 10

CHECK NUMBER OF 8 OZ
GLASSES OF WATER: ⬜ ⬜ ⬜ ⬜ ⬜ ⬜ ⬜ ⬜ ⬜ ⬜

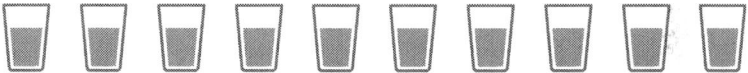

Time	Exercise	Amount

MOOD/CHALLENGES/NSV'S:

_____

_____

_____

HOURS FASTED BEFORE EATING: _____

HUNGER LEVEL:
1 2 3 4 5 6 7 8 9 10

M T W T F S S

DATE: _____

WEIGHT: _____

Time	Food/Beverage	Calories

STARTED NEW FAST AT: _____ / NA   ENERGY LEVEL: 1 2 3 4 5 6 7 8 9 10

CHECK NUMBER OF 8 OZ
GLASSES OF WATER:

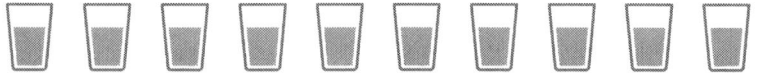

Time	Exercise	Amount

MOOD/CHALLENGES/NSV'S: _____
_____
_____
_____

DAY 68

M T W T F S S

Date: _____

Weight: _____

HOURS FASTED BEFORE EATING: _____

HUNGER LEVEL:
1 2 3 4 5 6 7 8 9 10

Time	Food/Beverage	Calories

STARTED NEW FAST AT: _____ / NA   ENERGY LEVEL: 1 2 3 4 5 6 7 8 9 10

CHECK NUMBER OF 8 OZ
GLASSES OF WATER:

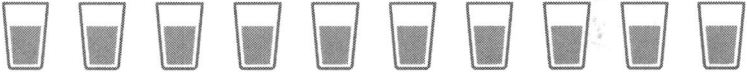

Time	Exercise	Amount

MOOD/CHALLENGES/NSV'S:

_____

_____

_____

HOURS FASTED BEFORE EATING: _____

HUNGER LEVEL:
1 2 3 4 5 6 7 8 9 10

M T W T F S S

DATE: _____

WEIGHT: _____

Time	Food/Beverage	Calories

STARTED NEW FAST AT: _____/ NA   ENERGY LEVEL: 1 2 3 4 5 6 7 8 9 10

CHECK NUMBER OF 8 OZ
GLASSES OF WATER:

Time	Exercise	Amount

MOOD/CHALLENGES/NSV'S:
_____
_____
_____
_____

DAY 70	M T W T F S S DATE: _____ WEIGHT: _____	HOURS FASTED BEFORE EATING: _____ HUNGER LEVEL: 1 2 3 4 5 6 7 8 9 10

Time	Food/Beverage	Calories

STARTED NEW FAST AT: _____ / NA   ENERGY LEVEL: 1 2 3 4 5 6 7 8 9 10

CHECK NUMBER OF 8 OZ GLASSES OF WATER:

Time	Exercise	Amount

MOOD/CHALLENGES/NSV'S:

_____
_____
_____

HOURS FASTED BEFORE EATING: _____

HUNGER LEVEL:

1 2 3 4 5 6 7 8 9 10

M T W T F S S

DATE: _____

WEIGHT: _____

DAY 71

Time	Food/Beverage	Calories

STARTED NEW FAST AT: _____ / NA   ENERGY LEVEL: 1 2 3 4 5 6 7 8 9 10

CHECK NUMBER OF 8 OZ GLASSES OF WATER:

Time	Exercise	Amount

MOOD/CHALLENGES/NSV'S: _____

_____

_____

_____

DAY 72

M T W T F S S

DATE: _____

WEIGHT: _____

HOURS FASTED BEFORE EATING: _____

HUNGER LEVEL:

1 2 3 4 5 6 7 8 9 10

Time	Food/Beverage	Calories

STARTED NEW FAST AT: _____ / NA   ENERGY LEVEL: 1 2 3 4 5 6 7 8 9 10

CHECK NUMBER OF 8 OZ GLASSES OF WATER:

Time	Exercise	Amount

MOOD/CHALLENGES/NSV'S:

_____

_____

_____

_____

HOURS FASTED BEFORE EATING: _____

HUNGER LEVEL:

1 2 3 4 5 6 7 8 9 10

M T W T F S S

DATE: _____

WEIGHT: _____

DAY
73

Time	Food/Beverage	Calories

STARTED NEW FAST AT: _____ / NA   ENERGY LEVEL: 1 2 3 4 5 6 7 8 9 10

CHECK NUMBER OF 8 OZ
GLASSES OF WATER:

Time	Exercise	Amount

MOOD/CHALLENGES/NSV'S: _____
_____
_____
_____

DAY 74

M T W T F S S

Date: _____

Weight: _____

HOURS FASTED BEFORE EATING: _____

HUNGER LEVEL:

1 2 3 4 5 6 7 8 9 10

Time	Food/Beverage	Calories

STARTED NEW FAST AT: _____ / NA   ENERGY LEVEL: 1 2 3 4 5 6 7 8 9 10

CHECK NUMBER OF 8 OZ
GLASSES OF WATER:

Time	Exercise	Amount

MOOD/CHALLENGES/NSV'S: _____
_____
_____
_____

HOURS FASTED BEFORE EATING: _____

HUNGER LEVEL:

1 2 3 4 5 6 7 8 9 10

M T W T F S S

DATE: _____

WEIGHT: _____

Time	Food/Beverage	Calories

STARTED NEW FAST AT: _____/ NA   ENERGY LEVEL: 1 2 3 4 5 6 7 8 9 10

CHECK NUMBER OF 8 OZ GLASSES OF WATER:

Time	Exercise	Amount

MOOD/CHALLENGES/NSV'S: _____

M T W T F S S

DATE: _____

WEIGHT: _____

HOURS FASTED BEFORE EATING: _____

HUNGER LEVEL:
1 2 3 4 5 6 7 8 9 10

Time	Food/Beverage	Calories

STARTED NEW FAST AT: _____ / NA   ENERGY LEVEL: 1 2 3 4 5 6 7 8 9 10

CHECK NUMBER OF 8 OZ
GLASSES OF WATER:

Time	Exercise	Amount

MOOD/CHALLENGES/NSV'S:

_____

_____

_____

HOURS FASTED BEFORE EATING: _____

HUNGER LEVEL:
1 2 3 4 5 6 7 8 9 10

M T W T F S S

DATE: _____

WEIGHT: _____

DAY
77

Time	Food/Beverage	Calories

STARTED NEW FAST AT: _____ / NA   ENERGY LEVEL: 1 2 3 4 5 6 7 8 9 10

CHECK NUMBER OF 8 OZ
GLASSES OF WATER:

Time	Exercise	Amount

MOOD/CHALLENGES/NSV'S: _____
_____
_____
_____

M T W T F S S

DATE: _____

WEIGHT: _____

HOURS FASTED BEFORE EATING: _____

HUNGER LEVEL:

1 2 3 4 5 6 7 8 9 10

Time	Food/Beverage	Calories

STARTED NEW FAST AT: _____ / NA   ENERGY LEVEL: 1 2 3 4 5 6 7 8 9 10

CHECK NUMBER OF 8 OZ
GLASSES OF WATER:

Time	Exercise	Amount

MOOD/CHALLENGES/NSV'S:

_____

_____

_____

HOURS FASTED BEFORE EATING: _____

HUNGER LEVEL:
1 2 3 4 5 6 7 8 9 10

M T W T F S S

DATE: _____

WEIGHT: _____

DAY 79

Time	Food/Beverage	Calories

STARTED NEW FAST AT: _____ / NA   ENERGY LEVEL: 1 2 3 4 5 6 7 8 9 10

CHECK NUMBER OF 8 OZ GLASSES OF WATER:

Time	Exercise	Amount

MOOD/CHALLENGES/NSV'S:
_____
_____
_____
_____

DAY 80

M T W T F S S

DATE: _____

WEIGHT: _____

HOURS FASTED BEFORE EATING: _____

HUNGER LEVEL:

1 2 3 4 5 6 7 8 9 10

Time	Food/Beverage	Calories

STARTED NEW FAST AT: _____/ NA   ENERGY LEVEL: 1 2 3 4 5 6 7 8 9 10

CHECK NUMBER OF 8 OZ
GLASSES OF WATER:

Time	Exercise	Amount

MOOD/CHALLENGES/NSV'S:

_____

_____

_____

HOURS FASTED BEFORE EATING: _____

HUNGER LEVEL:

1 2 3 4 5 6 7 8 9 10

M T W T F S S

DATE: _____

WEIGHT: _____

DAY 81

Time	Food/Beverage	Calories

STARTED NEW FAST AT: _____/ NA   ENERGY LEVEL: 1 2 3 4 5 6 7 8 9 10

CHECK NUMBER OF 8 OZ GLASSES OF WATER:

Time	Exercise	Amount

MOOD/CHALLENGES/NSV'S: _____

_____

_____

_____

DAY 82	M T W T F S S

DATE: _____

WEIGHT: _____

HOURS FASTED BEFORE EATING: _____

HUNGER LEVEL:

1 2 3 4 5 6 7 8 9 10

Time	Food/Beverage	Calories

STARTED NEW FAST AT: _____ / NA   ENERGY LEVEL: 1 2 3 4 5 6 7 8 9 10

CHECK NUMBER OF 8 OZ
GLASSES OF WATER:

Time	Exercise	Amount

MOOD/CHALLENGES/NSV'S: _____

_____

_____

_____

HOURS FASTED BEFORE EATING: _____

HUNGER LEVEL:

1 2 3 4 5 6 7 8 9 10

M T W T F S S

DATE: _____

WEIGHT: _____

DAY 83

Time	Food/Beverage	Calories

STARTED NEW FAST AT: _____/ NA   ENERGY LEVEL: 1 2 3 4 5 6 7 8 9 10

CHECK NUMBER OF 8 OZ
GLASSES OF WATER:

Time	Exercise	Amount

MOOD/CHALLENGES/NSV'S:

_____

_____

_____

DAY 84

M T W T F S S

Date: _____

Weight: _____

HOURS FASTED BEFORE EATING: _____

HUNGER LEVEL:
1 2 3 4 5 6 7 8 9 10

Time	Food/Beverage	Calories

STARTED NEW FAST AT: _____ / NA   ENERGY LEVEL: 1 2 3 4 5 6 7 8 9 10

CHECK NUMBER OF 8 OZ GLASSES OF WATER:

Time	Exercise	Amount

MOOD/CHALLENGES/NSV'S:

_____

_____

_____

HOURS FASTED BEFORE EATING: _____

HUNGER LEVEL:
1 2 3 4 5 6 7 8 9 10

M T W T F S S

DATE: _____

WEIGHT: _____

DAY
85

Time	Food/Beverage	Calories

STARTED NEW FAST AT: _____/ NA   ENERGY LEVEL: 1 2 3 4 5 6 7 8 9 10

CHECK NUMBER OF 8 OZ
GLASSES OF WATER:

Time	Exercise	Amount

MOOD/CHALLENGES/NSV'S: _____
_____
_____
_____

M T W T F S S

DATE: _____

WEIGHT: _____

HOURS FASTED BEFORE EATING: _____

HUNGER LEVEL:

1 2 3 4 5 6 7 8 9 10

Time	Food/Beverage	Calories

STARTED NEW FAST AT: _____ / NA   ENERGY LEVEL: 1 2 3 4 5 6 7 8 9 10

CHECK NUMBER OF 8 OZ GLASSES OF WATER:

Time	Exercise	Amount

MOOD/CHALLENGES/NSV'S:

_____

_____

_____

HOURS FASTED BEFORE EATING: _____

HUNGER LEVEL:

1 2 3 4 5 6 7 8 9 10

M T W T F S S

DATE: _____

WEIGHT: _____

DAY
87

Time	Food/Beverage	Calories

STARTED NEW FAST AT: _____ / NA   ENERGY LEVEL: 1 2 3 4 5 6 7 8 9 10

CHECK NUMBER OF 8 OZ
GLASSES OF WATER:

Time	Exercise	Amount

MOOD/CHALLENGES/NSV'S:

DAY 88	M T W T F S S Date: _____ Weight: _____	Hours Fasted Before Eating: _____ Hunger Level: 1 2 3 4 5 6 7 8 9 10

Time	Food/Beverage	Calories

Started New Fast At: _____ / NA   Energy Level: 1 2 3 4 5 6 7 8 9 10

Check Number of 8 Oz Glasses of Water:

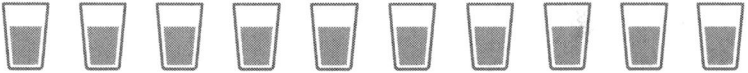

Time	Exercise	Amount

Mood/Challenges/NSV's:

_____
_____
_____
_____

HOURS FASTED BEFORE EATING: _____

HUNGER LEVEL:
1 2 3 4 5 6 7 8 9 10

M T W T F S S

DATE: _____

WEIGHT: _____

DAY 89

Time	Food/Beverage	Calories

STARTED NEW FAST AT: _____/ NA   ENERGY LEVEL: 1 2 3 4 5 6 7 8 9 10

CHECK NUMBER OF 8 OZ
GLASSES OF WATER:

Time	Exercise	Amount

MOOD/CHALLENGES/NSV'S: _____
_____
_____
_____

M T W T F S · S

DATE: _____

WEIGHT: _____

HOURS FASTED BEFORE EATING: _____

HUNGER LEVEL:

1 2 3 4 5 6 7 8 9 10

Time	Food/Beverage	Calories

STARTED NEW FAST AT: _____ / NA   ENERGY LEVEL: 1 2 3 4 5 6 7 8 9 10

CHECK NUMBER OF 8 OZ
GLASSES OF WATER:

Time	Exercise	Amount

MOOD/CHALLENGES/NSV'S:

_____

_____

_____

Made in the USA
Las Vegas, NV
13 November 2021